TABLE OF CONTENTS

Introduction

Human body basics………..

In the story of creation we gather that man was formed using the earth or soil then God breathed His spirit into man and he became a living being. In the creation process of nature such as people, plants and animals, God installed reproduction and repair wisdom or instructions. Since then people, plants and animals multiply through reproduction and self heal or self repair as and when necessary. This aspect of self reproduction and self repair ensured that God did not have to keep recreating or repairing injuries to living things.

Man is made of flesh and blood. Believe it or not, the substances that form the liver, the skin, the hair and the kidneys are minerals and elements found in the earth whose formula and combination is known to God only and a mystery to man. The human body contains wisdom for regeneration whenever there is a wound or defect. It does this using resources available to it within the body system. If one does not drink enough water to cleanse off toxins and assist with internal body processes, the internal water becomes dirty and that same dirty water shall be used to regenerate body cells when the need arises. Cell regeneration wisdom and instructions installed at creation will not stop functioning because there are inadequate resources or unclean environment. It simply makes use of what is available to execute its mandate.

Adequate clean water and an internal environment with abundant resources for cell regeneration and repair ensures a faster regeneration process which results in healthy body cells and ultimately a very efficient and effective body part resulting in overall quicker healing for the whole body while an unclean environment results in a slower or longer regeneration and healing process and a weak, less effective and inefficient body part.

When a plant does not have enough water its cells shrivel and this is evidenced by wilting. If the water situation around the plant does not improve, the plant eventually dries up and dies. Similarly humans and animals go through the same process. It sets off as a feeling of weakness then develops into lying down and not being able to move or carry out any activities and may even lead to hospitalisation. If the situation is not resolved, this eventually leads to loss of life.

People who live in hot climates consume more water than those in cool or cold climates on a daily basis. This is because through sweating and perspiration, water is lost from the human body a lot faster and needs more frequent replenishment. At any point and time the body should have a balance of the water it carries internally against its external environment.

As with water, the mineral and nutrient content within the body should also be enough to cope with the stress, weather and routine daily activities the body goes through. When such a scenario exists, a state of wellness and well being prevails in a person. Absence of that balance initially sets off a craving which if not resolved then develops into discomfort or restlessness. This restlessness and discomfort if not addressed will further develop into body weakness and illness as resources continue to deplete.

Cell, tissue and organ deterioration and eventual damage due to failure to address the lack of resources required, develops in phases. The situation develops from little easy to address and reversible damage, then to moderate damage which may take a bit of a while to resolve and then further into a bad situation where extensive damage which will take a while and require more effort and dedication to resolve. In worst case scenarios, the situation becomes unresolvable and the organ eventually stops functioning and may need replacement. In cases where organ replacement is impossible it eventually leads to death.

Failure of one internal organ to function can result in death because all body organs depend on each other for optimum performance. Internal organs are each other's bridges. They connect one part of the body's internal environment to another. If the bridge malfunctions, all internal organs are affected and if it completely breaks down a section of the body completely disconnects from the other. This cuts off supply of resources needed for the function and survival of other organs leading to eventual shut down of the whole system which we call death.

External body organs rely on the well being and optimum functioning of the internal body system. It is possible for somebody not to have legs, hands or eyes but still be able to live normally using artificial systems around them to cope. The same cannot be said for the heart, liver, kidneys and all other internal organs. Malfunction or absolute dysfunction of any one of these will result in the whole system packing up and being sent back to mother earth 6 feet below the earth surface.

Chapter 1

Plant basics....

All plants retrieve nutrients from the earth or soil to use together with other atmospheric components like carbon dioxide and sunlight for their growth, survival and reproduction. Each plant has its own set of wisdom or instructions which makes it unique and different from other plants. The uniqueness is visibly evident in the size of the plant, the shape and colour of the leaves,the fruits and the plant's life span.

An orchard can have a variety of trees i.e. a guava tree, lemon tree, avocado tree, mango tree, peach tree or any fruit tree growing in the same environment. Likewise a vegetable garden can also have tomato plants, potato plants, spinach, carrots, cabbages, kale, covo, egg plants, leeks, onions etc all growing under the same weather conditions, same soil structure, texture and earth minerals, elements and components yet they will produce different fruits and vegetables which will be ready for consumption in different seasons. This is because each plant carries in it wisdom and instructions to retrieve particular minerals and nutrients in particular quantities and combinations from the same earth and process them over a certain period of time to then produce a particular fruit or vegetable in a particular season. Different fruit trees and vegetables will flower and produce different fruits or vegetable leaves in different seasons though they are in the same environment and growing under similar conditions. How is this so?

The plant system through its roots retrieves or absorbs nutrients and minerals then transport them up the stem to the branches and leaves which then process food for the plant processes enabling them to produce unique fruits and vegetables guided by the naturally installed wisdom or instructions. In simple terms the same mineral elements and nutrients are used by different plants in different combinations to bring out the different outcomes in the form of fruits and vegetables.

Fruit trees and vegetables produce seed either carried inside the fruit or in a pod or some protective casing. The seed contains wisdom and instructions which, when planted, subjected or exposed to conducive conditions bring forth another plant of the same type.

Why do different fruits or plants carry varying quantities of seeds? This is God or Creator order and a clear message and direction that the plant fruits, leaves etc should be consumed, replanted and reproduced at a rate equivalent or directly proportional to the number of seeds the fruit or the plant carries. Why else would God put more seeds in one plant and less in another?

Different plants have different life spans. The plants with shorter life spans generally carry more seed while those with longer life spans carry moderate amounts of seed with some fruits like avocado, apricots and plums carrying only one seed. These variations in lifespan and seed content indicate the rate or frequency at which the plant leaves or fruit should be consumed and seeds replanted for reproduction.

Trees are bigger and taller in size with longer life spans while vegetables are generally smaller and shorter with shorter life spans. Trees take years to mature and bear fruit and can live for decades and even centuries in some instances for example the baobab tree. The baobab fruit carries a significantly large amount of seed compared to other fruit trees. The fruit and its leaves are highly nutritious and filled with loads of vitamins. This is a typical example of a tree whose products should be taken in large quantities because of their nutritional value and should also multiply to cater for human demands.

Vegetable plants generally carry more seed for reproduction while trees carry less seed. They usually mature in 90 days or more depending on type of vegetable and its life cycle. Some vegetable plants are seasonal while others are not. They can be replanted for reproduction at the end of their life cycle.

Low lying plants tend to have more seed because they are also largely consumed by animals that creep, crawl and walk the ground. Animals like rabbits, goats, sheep etc may not be able to climb up trees but can access the low lying plants. The abundance of seed in such plants is to cater for the high demand from both people and animals. There should be reproduction of such plants in volumes in direct proportion to the seed content. As plant height increases some living things because of height disadvantage are excluded from consuming fruits of such plants. Such plants tend to have seeds for reproduction in moderation.

When a fruit is in formation, it feeds off nutrients from the leaves of the plant. Orange tree leaves will give the same benefits that oranges give because whatever is contained in an orange comes from the leaves. The leaves also contain the instructions and nutrient combinations that give oranges their colour and they release to the fruit the nutrients for the process. Fruits contain easily and readily digestible nutrients and sugars.

Leaves contain the same nutrients in slightly more complex forms such that they have to be taken through a process of breaking down complex nutrient structures so that the become soluble. They are usually steeped in boiled or very hot water to breakdown the complex structures so that they become soluble and are taken as teas. The tender or new leaves of a tree are thinner, lighter in colour and the nutrients in them are more soluble and easily retrieved.

The older the leaves grow the more food is stored in them and the more complex the nutrient structures. They become thicker and darker in colour as a sign of the richer food stocks. The nutrients are less soluble and the leaves need to be boiled to break the complex structures into substances that are easily digested and absorbed by the human body. They are usually taken up as teas.

The barks, stems and roots of the plants will also carry even more complex structures of the same substances found in the fruits and leaves because they also serve as nutrient storage sites.

The leaves of a plant also known as the kitchen of the plant is where plant food is made. When leaves are shed off or eaten or taken off by other living things for whatever reason the plant would be expected to die. Seasons will wipe out all leaves from a tree and leave absolutely nothing but the tree will still not die. After cutting off a large part of a tree, it will bud and grow again as long as the roots are alive underground. All this happens because whenever there is a shortage on the plant the stem and roots release the nutrients stored in them for the leaf regeneration process and any other processes the plant needs to carry out. These stored nutrients are broken down by the plant into simpler structures for the use of the plant by small protein substances called enzymes. They are then released into other parts of the plant based on the same wisdom and instructions that specifies the unique combination of minerals, elements and nutrients.

Having understood this, we see that the whole plant from the root to its tip contains the same nutrients in varying complexities. It can therefore be concluded that in the absence of fruits and leaves people can still benefit from the roots, bark and stems. These however have to boiled longer than leaves are boiled so that the complex structures in them are broken down to release nutrients stored in them into forms that are easy to digest, easy to absorb and use by the human body system. The nutrients stored in barks, stems and roots are however more concentrated since they are storage sites.

Chapter 2

The co-relation between people, plants and animals…..

Each second that passes, a zillion chemical processes take place all over the whole body. Body processes grow the body, repair or heal, regenerate, digest, remove toxins, absorb nutrients, create energy etc for use by cells as they carry out body processes and for other internal and external practical body activities such as working, walking, talking, seeing, hearing, cooking, thinking, laughing etc. Body cells use nutrients, minerals, vitamins, water etc to make all these things happen. For the liver to function at its best it requires certain minerals, vitamins and nutrients in certain quantities or proportions and combinations. The same applies to the kidneys, the heart, the spleen, the brain etc. Each body part has its own specific combination of minerals, nutrients and vitamins required for it to operate at its optimum capacity as required by the body. Body requirements vary according to gender, age, body weight, height and daily activities. A pregnant woman will demand more nutrients and minerals as compared to one who isn't and a man who does a lot of exercising, working out or hard physical work will demand some substances more than one who does not.

Weather conditions and external environment also exert their own pressure and also influence the rate at which the body uses up nutrients and minerals in the body. If living under hot weather conditions where a lot of sweating takes place as the body tries to cool itself, salts are lost through the sweating process.

Any compromise in the quantities of minerals, nutrients and vitamins required by any body organ to function efficiently and effectively will result in that organ not operating at the required level and that in turn will affect the other body organs and the body system as a whole. For instance if the body does not have enough salts or sugars for the efficient functioning of the heart, the heart will not operate at its required capacity. A craving for salty or sweet food is set off. Meanwhile this means that not enough oxygen will reach all body parts and the body feels weak. This is because the effective and efficient functioning of individual internal organs has been affected and ultimately the whole body. Prolonged failure to address the issue may result in one fainting, shortness of breath and may need to be connected to an oxygen supply while the issue gets addressed.

Likewise excess nutrients, minerals and salts will result in toxicity of the environment the body organ is operating in. Too much of a good thing can become poisonous, lead to illness and even death. Salt makes food taste good, however too much of it makes the same food inedible and a danger to the body. The same applies with the sugar, oil, zinc, magnesium content in the body among other things required by the body. Excess of anything will affect the cells, organs and the body as a whole. It will also result in feelings of discomfort and un-wellness and if not addressed illness and ultimately death. The body however has God installed wisdom, instructions and mechanisms to remove any excess substances and maintain the correct balance of nutrients, minerals and vitamins.

As discussed earlier a state of well being is achieved when there are adequate amounts of minerals, nutrients, water content etc for the optimum functioning of the body organs according to their individual requirements and ultimately the body as a whole. This is why nowadays upon visiting a medical facility for treatment they initially run blood tests to check for blood content. This helps in isolating the root causes of un-wellness and assist in prescribing the correct treatment for the body to be restored to normal function and a feeling of wellness.

For one to maintain a situation of consistent wellness there should constant and consistent replenishment of required substances through breathing, eating and drinking. The body cells and organs use whatever is taken in for their processes and reject what they do not require. If a required resource is missing the body places a demand through a craving.

The relationship between man and plants is that the fruit trees and vegetable plants through their leaves, fruits, stems, bark etc directly replenish the body system of required substances. How does that happen? As discussed earlier plant wisdom makes it take up from the earth certain or particular minerals in unique proportions and combinations that then result in the formation of a particular fruit unique to that particular plant. That combination of minerals, elements, nutrients and salts is carried in the fruit, leaves and rest of the plant. On eating that fruit or vegetable all its resource wealth is released into the body's systems and enriches the body with its contents. This release supplies the body cells and organs with the resources needed for continuous day to day healthy functioning.

Likewise the roots, stems and barks of the plant contain same nutrients as fruits and leaves but in more concentrated forms as discussed earlier. Their consumption should therefore not be at the same rate as that of fruits and leaves. Unlike fruits they are not sweet and do not have a pleasant taste. In most cases they are bitter. The concentrated versions of nutrients stored in roots, stems and barks also have capacity to address or cure some conditions and ailments in humans that low concentrations in fruits and leaves may not be able to rapidly address.

God through His wisdom created seasons and along with those seasons vegetables and fruits to replenish the body of lost or needed nutrients to cope with the demands and stresses that arise due to weather conditions, normal daily activities or unique seasonal activities. It is by design that a particular tree will yield a particular fruit in a particular season. The reason being that, the tree has been God programmed to take up from the earth or soil certain combinations and proportions of minerals, elements and nutrients and process them over a particular period before packaging them for distribution to man as attractive and delicious fruits. Mineral salts, nutrients and vitamin deficiencies can also arise as a result of previous season's activities and weather conditions which will have used up resources needed by the body to cope with current season demands.

Besides being seasonal, plants are also geographical and climactic. God has set up earth that certain plants are found in certain areas depending on the climatic or weather conditions. A baobab tree is very prominent in areas with high temperatures and almost non existent in cool climates. This has to do with the particular nutrient needs and requirements of the people living in those climate conditions. In some cases you will find variations of the same plant family growing in different weather conditions for example sweet apple or graviola or soursop in West Africa is the equivalent of custard apple in southern Africa. There are some plants that will thrive under any conditions but may taste different depending on the environment they developed under.

Water melons for instance are seasonally available. They are a summer fruit where temperatures are high. They are known as hydrating fruits because they have high water content which when consumed replenishes the body's water levels. Lycopene the red pigment or colour in water melons protects the body against damage caused by pesticides, herbicides etc which are largely used in summer as it is the planting season because of the rains. Its also an antioxidant which protects the body from damage caused by free radicals hence protecting against cancer. Lycopene improves heart health and prevents against sunburn. The nutritional value of lycopene specifically targets the well being of the heart. The proper or efficient function of the heart ensures blood is pumped to the whole body so that nutrients, water and oxygen reach all parts of the body. People are usually very active and up and about in summer which places a higher\demand on the heart's function.

The number of seeds in a fruit is a direct indication of how much of it to consume in any given season. More seeds mean more of that fruit should be consumed, moderate number indicates moderate consumption while one seed means regular eating. One should aim to eat all the fruits available in a season according to the seed prescribed frequencies. Every fruit has its own major unique role which other fruits may not satisfy.

Each fruit and each plant almost always contains a certain amount of all required nutrients by the body. They however carry dominant nutrients and give the fruit or vegetable its dominant function. This effectively means each plant has dominant or main functions and secondary functions. It also further means that functions and benefits from fruits and vegetables never exist in isolation. The other present nutrients and elements still provide their benefits to the body even in their lesser quantities. These will however not be adequate to meet the body's demands or requirements of the particular substance and problems caused by deficiencies of such substances will manifest still manifest though not in a devastating way. That is why it is therefore necessary to consume all fruits and vegetables available in a season. It is natural and normal to like or favour a certain fruit or vegetable over another. Too much of one thing though will not be good or healthy for the body.

It is important to note that a craving is different from a liking of a particular fruit or vegetable. A craving comes unexpectedly and creates a desire to consume a particular thing which is then quenched by consuming that particular thing which one may not ordinarily like, while liking is having an interest to eat a particular thing because it is pleasant. Liking makes one buy a thing even when they did not really feel hungry or a burning desire to consume it.

If plants retrieve nutrients from the earth or soil and can supply the body with everything needed then how does meat fit into the picture? Animals eat the leaves and fruits of plants. They eat the unprocessed leaves and have digestive systems that process and reprocess the difficult to digest leaves and plant parts till they are soluble and can be absorbed into their blood stream and body system. Cows for instance have four stomachs and they chew the curd meaning processed food will come back by reverse peristalsis, gets processed again and goes back into the stomachs until it gets fully reprocessed and can be absorbed by their body system.

The nutrients from the digested food are absorbed into the blood stream and transported to all the body cells and parts of the particular animal. We have all witnessed very healthy looking cows, goats, zebras etc that feed on just plant matter. Some make a very captivating and pleasant sight. Animals like humans also process and store in their bodies what is contained in the plants and build up healthy, fleshy organs with shiny attractive coats. People then slaughter these animals and consume their juicy, tasty and fleshy meat. The meat is very healthy and contains nutrients beneficial to the human body. This then leaves the argument that people eat meat as a main protein source. Goats, sheep, cows, zebras and many other herbivores do not consume meat but still develop healthy, fleshy tasty organs from consuming plants.

It has always been recommended to consume animals that eat plants i.e. herbivores against animals that consume other animals i.e. carnivores. When a carnivore eats a herbivore then a person eats the carnivore, the person is now third in the nutrient benefit chain. Original nutrients were processed and absorbed by the herbivore meaning it would have used up the nutrients it absorbed from the plant food. The carnivorous animal therefore benefits more from eating the herbivore. This then compromises the benefits that can be accrued by a person through eating a carnivorous animal.

Chapter 3

Completing the cycle….

All nature is made up of nutrients from the earth or soil and on dying or disposal it buried back into the ground or earth where it decomposes and disintegrates into the original small little individual selves. Upon disintegrating they enrich the earth or soil with nutrients they carried in them initially absorbed from the ground. These can then be re-absorbed by plants. They are a ready source of high nutritional value and content needed by the plant and they make the plant grow into a very healthy plant.

The process of setting up a compost involves loading it up with a layer of dead, dry plant material such as branches and leaves, then adding a layer of soil and more dead plant material and remains from food stuffs, kitchen waste like egg shells, banana peels, chicken feathers, meat that has gone bad, potato peels etc and add another layer of soil on top. The number of layers depends on one's personal preference or interest depending on what they want to achieve. It may also be influenced by possible availability of soil and kitchen waste, garden waste, weeds, dead plant material etc. Some people actually sell compost. After a while all those things that were being added to the compost totally disintegrate and can no longer be separately identified. They all looks the same as soil except with a richer texture. The same happens when animals or humans die. They rot and disintegrate into their initial small particles and re-unite with the rest of the soil or earth. After a while everything looks just like the soil. Upon taking that enriched soil where some stuff which used to be living matter has disintegrated and adding it onto the ground where a living plant is growing, there will be a boost in the plant growth and healthy appearance.

Animal waste on the other hand is also plant material that has been processed by the animal in its digestive system and removed from the body for varying reasons such as being indigestible or excess and not required. Though it is waste it still contains some of the elements, minerals etc that were initially extracted from the earth. Likewise if added to a plant or soil around a plant, it results in a boost in growth and the health of the plant. That is why animal waste is good manure or food for the plant. It is a ready source of nutrients.

The reason why dead plant and animal matter and waste causes a boost or positive change in the growth and appearance of a plant is because nutrients that the roots would ordinarily grow in search of either along the ground or deep into the ground will have been supplied through the dead matter and waste. It becomes readily available.

Ever wondered why plant roots bend, twist and turn into different directions giving them varying unique shapes? This happens as the roots develop and grow in the direction in which the nutrients or water the plant needs and seek are in abundance. This behaviour is similar to that of a craving in a human being or animal. Plants have an inbuilt mechanism that makes them grow towards where what they require is. A part of a root my become thicker than one before it or after it, because at the point where it is thick, there was an abundance of resources it required that boosted its development. If the plant roots do not find required nutrients signs of poor growth and ill health begin to manifest in the shoot of the plant. The shoot is the part of the plant that is above the ground.

When a woman is pregnant, she has unique food cravings which arise due to a demand by the growing foetus in her womb. Satisfying the food cravings ensures required nutrients reach the foetus for a healthy development.

Bones do not easily disintegrate like flesh does. However after millions and millions of years upon continuous addition of soil on bones, pressure and temperatures increase upon them underground, they eventually disintegrate and convert to fossils from which fossil fuels are derived. When such a process takes place on dry ground coal and gas are formed and when it happens under the oceans and seas or water bodies, oils from which petrols, diesel and other such oil products are then processed, are formed for use by people and for industrial activities.

It can therefore be concluded that man, animals and plants are unique combinations of earth minerals, elements and components all retrieved from the earth or the ground and developed or brought together using God wisdom and instructions. They live and die and go back to the ground where they are reabsorbed by plants and processed into combinations that bring out edible leaves and fruits for animals and people. Trees also produce oxygen required by people and animals to live. In the absence of oxygen death becomes the status. People and animals release carbon dioxide which the plants need. Absence of carbon dioxide results in the death of plants. People, plants and animals are earth or soil expressed in unique ways as a result of unique mineral combinations and life is a continuous, interdependent, ongoing cycle of nutrients made up of the earth or soil, people, plants and animals.

Chapter 4

A reconciliation of facts

Plants are herbs and herbs are plants. They were created by God with a mandate which is largely for the well being of people and animals. All plants release oxygen as a waste. People and animals need this oxygen for survival. Plants absorb carbon dioxide which is a waste from human beings and use the carbon dioxide for its biological processes. If carbon dioxide is not absorbed by the plants, the air will become toxic and people and animals will all die.

In addition to oxygen production each plant has its own unique functions. Some have beautiful flowers that decorate the earth, others give a pleasant smell, most of them make delicious healing teas and they all provide cools shades when its hot. Some produce fruit which is food for both people and animals. Animals eat the leaves of plants and at times the stems and roots too.

Eating the meat of an animal that has eaten the leaves of a plant is not an evil or ungodly act. Eating fruit of a plant is also not an evil or ungodly act. As explained in earlier chapters the fruit actually develops using nutrients supplied through the leaves.

People, plants and animals are dependent on each other for survival and form part of the cycle of nature. None of the components of the nature cycle is evil. Consumption of leaves, stems or roots and even flowers of a plant is in no way evil. They are all formed and develop using nutrients and elements from the earth or soil. If any of that should be considered evil or ungodly then it makes the soil or earth evil because all of nature is nutrients, elements and minerals coming from the earth and assembled in different and unique combinations to bring out the different things on earth. People, plants and animals are there for each other's well being using the earth or soil as a source of resources. It is a God designed natural survival system.

When one falls ill from reasons expressed above nature is the next best thing to heal them. If diet and nutrition are not well managed in relation to nature problems arise. If addressed early then they are easily resolvable. If left to deteriorate then hospitalisation will be the only way to go where higher level intensive treatment is administered.

Correct eating pattern should be the first port of staying well and healing. Have you noticed that when a person is unwell they are largely fed fruits and vegetable broth. Vegetable broth is made from different vegetables and almost always results in an unwell person regaining their appetite and energy. Against this background it is encouraged to love your fruits, vegetables, spices, herbal teas in their varieties. Consume them in their seasons in appropriate quantities and you will maintain top notch health and may never have need to take drugs for anything because this basically keeps sickness and disease away.

There are beliefs among some religious sects that consuming herbs or leaves of plants is diabolic and a reflection of one's lack of faith, trust, not being very prayerful or weak belief in God and that God can heal them.

Without foregoing the supernatural power of God through prayer, it is evident that God already set up natural healing processes when he created nature. It is by being responsible and taking care of the body which is the temple of the Holy Ghost by eating properly that a maintains good health. A person cannot continue to be irresponsible and practice bad eating habits and continuously be praying and asking God to heal them. It is not sustainable. Some sects believe that only water that has been prayed for heals. Water is just part of what the body needs. It does not have the capacity to address that which should be addressed by other minerals and nutrients from the earth. Water has its limits.

It is therefore certainly not evil or diabolic to consume the leaves of plants. If consuming a banana or a mango is not evil then consuming mango or banana leaves cannot be evil. From the first chapter we note that whatever is in a banana or mango actually came from the leaves and is found in the leaves and the rest of the plant too. In the same breath if it is not evil to consume the flesh or meat of an animal that ate leaves of a plant then it cannot be evil for a person to consume the same leaves directly.

The pharmaceutical industries have over the years understood the plant system and the healing nature of plants. Through chemical processes they conducted laboratory analyses of the constituents of plants to discover the dominant chemical structures and components that effected the healing aspect in plants.

They then sought to replicate the plant systems
process and started producing drugs en mass. They
came up with systems of extracting nutrients and
minerals from the earth and processing them in a
laboratories and mass producing in factories. It is in a
way similar to what a tree does.

The major differences are that in the process of
extracting the required substances and separating
them from other unrequired substances from the soil,
they use chemicals which may be harsh but still bring
them to process a replica of the desired substance.
Plants in contrast use pure naturally God installed
wisdom, instructions and mechanisms and have a way
of extracting the required elements from the earth and
filtering out what is not required. Plants have a full
combination and complement of minerals and
nutrients while pills are largely usually made using
the main active ingredient. An active ingredient is the
identified dominant nutrient in a plant. For instance a
moringa leaf can address many health issues. The
same leaf can be processed to extract oil from it
which can still address some health issues and the
cake that is left after extracting the oil will also still
be able to address health issues. This means the whole
moringa leaf has components which can be separated
and still be effective in their isolated versions. The
isolated versions though can never be more powerful
than the whole unprocessed moringa leaf. From this
we can conclude it is better and more beneficial to
maintain health by consuming various plant
components as compared to then seek healing from
drugs.

The Conclusion...........

Without knowledge and understanding of what constitutes the body, it is very difficult to successfully manage, maintain and uphold its well being. It either gets damaged or destroyed and its life span compromised from lack of knowledge. From this day make a concerted effort to know your body, listen to it, feel it, understand it and take good care of it. Make an effort to understand how you relate to nature and commune with with it. If that is diligently done then a long healthy life is almost certain.